TABLE OF CONTENTS

INTRODUCTION

Pregnancy, often hailed as a period of joy and anticipation, can also bring about a myriad of challenges, one of the most common being pregnancy sickness. Characterized by nausea, vomiting, and general discomfort, pregnancy sickness affects a significant proportion of expectant mothers worldwide. Despite its prevalence, the management of pregnancy sickness remains a complex and often perplexing aspect of maternal healthcare.

In recent years, the field of healthcare has witnessed a remarkable transformation propelled by advancements in artificial intelligence (AI) technologies. From diagnostic tools to treatment algorithms, AI has emerged as a powerful ally in the quest for more personalized and effective healthcare solutions. Nowhere is this potential more apparent than in the realm of pregnancy sickness management.

The book you hold in your hands, "Utilizing Artificial Intelligence for Personalized Management of Pregnancy Sickness: Challenges, Opportunities, and Future Directions," seeks to explore the intersection of AI and maternal healthcare with a specific focus on pregnancy sickness. Within these pages, we embark on a journey to understand the multifaceted nature of pregnancy sickness, the evolving landscape of AI in healthcare, and the promise it holds for personalized management strategies tailored to the unique needs of each expectant mother.

Our exploration begins by delving into the nuances of pregnancy sickness its symptoms, prevalence, and the profound impact it can have on the physical and emotional well-being of pregnant individuals. We unravel the complexities inherent in its management, confronting the variability of symptoms, the limitations of existing treatment modalities, and the persistent gaps in our understanding of its underlying mechanisms.

Against this backdrop, we turn our gaze to the transformative potential of artificial intelligence. We witness its capacity to analyze vast troves of data, discern patterns amidst complexity, and generate insights that elude conventional approaches. Through AI-driven decision support systems and personalized treatment algorithms, we envision a future where pregnancy sickness management is not only more effective but also more tailored to the unique needs and preferences of each patient.

Yet, as we embark on this journey of innovation and discovery, we are mindful of the challenges that lie ahead. Ethical considerations loom large as we navigate the terrain of patient privacy, data security, and algorithmic fairness. We confront the inherent biases embedded within AI systems and strive to forge a path towards more equitable and inclusive healthcare solutions.

As we traverse the pages of this book, we encounter real-world case studies, research findings, and insights gleaned from the front lines of maternal healthcare. We uncover success stories and lessons learned, charting a course towards a future where pregnancy sickness is not merely managed but truly understood and empowered by the transformative potential of artificial intelligence.

In the chapters that follow, we invite you to join us on this voyage of exploration and discovery. Together, let us unravel the mysteries of pregnancy sickness, harness the power of artificial intelligence, and chart a course towards a future where every expectant mother receives the personalized care and support she deserves.

Welcome to the forefront of maternal healthcare innovation. Welcome to "Utilizing Artificial Intelligence for Personalized Management of Pregnancy Sickness: Challenges, Opportunities, and Future Directions."

Overview of Pregnancy Sickness

Pregnancy, often heralded as a time of joy and anticipation, can also bring about a range of physical and emotional challenges for expectant mothers. Among these challenges, pregnancy sickness stands as one of the most common and often debilitating conditions experienced during gestation. Characterized by symptoms such as nausea, vomiting, and general discomfort, pregnancy sickness can significantly impact the quality of life and overall well-being of pregnant individuals.

In this section of "Utilizing Artificial Intelligence for Personalized Management of Pregnancy Sickness: Challenges, Opportunities, and Future Directions," we embark on a comprehensive exploration of pregnancy sickness, seeking to understand its multifaceted nature, prevalence, impact, and management strategies.

We begin by defining pregnancy sickness and delineating its various manifestations, ranging from mild queasiness to severe and persistent vomiting, known clinically as hyperemesis gravidarum. By elucidating the spectrum of symptoms and their potential impact on maternal health, we aim to provide readers with a nuanced understanding of the condition's complexity.

Next, we delve into the prevalence of pregnancy sickness, highlighting its ubiquity across diverse populations and cultural contexts. Through epidemiological data and research findings, we illuminate the widespread nature of pregnancy sickness and underscore the importance of developing effective management strategies to support expectant mothers through this challenging period.

Moreover, we explore the potential causes and triggers of pregnancy sickness, acknowledging the role of hormonal fluctuations, genetic predispositions, dietary factors, and psychosocial stressors in contributing to its onset and severity. By unraveling the underlying mechanisms of pregnancy sickness, we aim to foster a deeper appreciation of its etiology and inform the development of targeted interventions.

As we navigate the landscape of pregnancy sickness management, we confront the limitations of existing treatment modalities and the need for more personalized and evidence-based approaches. From dietary modifications and lifestyle interventions to pharmacological therapies and complementary modalities, we examine the array of options available to healthcare providers and expectant mothers alike.

Throughout this exploration, we remain cognizant of the profound impact that pregnancy sickness can have on the physical, emotional, and social well-being of pregnant individuals. By elevating the voices and experiences of those affected by pregnancy sickness, we seek to foster empathy, understanding, and solidarity within the broader healthcare community.

In the chapters that follow, we embark on a journey to uncover the potential of artificial intelligence in revolutionizing the personalized management of pregnancy sickness. By harnessing the power of data analytics, machine learning algorithms, and personalized medicine approaches, we aspire to redefine the standard of care for expectant mothers facing the challenges of pregnancy sickness.

Importance of Personalized Management

In the realm of maternal healthcare, personalized management holds profound significance, particularly when addressing the complexities of pregnancy sickness. As we navigate the myriad factors contributing to this condition, from hormonal fluctuations to genetic predispositions, the one-size-fits-all approach to treatment falls short in meeting the diverse needs and preferences of expectant mothers. In this section of "Utilizing Artificial Intelligence for Personalized Management of Pregnancy

Sickness: Challenges, Opportunities, and Future Directions," we explore the importance of personalized management strategies in optimizing maternal health outcomes.

Tailored Interventions: Pregnancy sickness manifests uniquely in each individual, with symptoms varying in severity, duration, and response to treatment. By adopting a personalized approach to management, healthcare providers can tailor interventions to address the specific needs and preferences of expectant mothers, optimizing treatment efficacy and patient satisfaction.

Minimization of Adverse Effects: Traditional treatment modalities for pregnancy sickness, such as pharmacological therapies, may pose risks of adverse effects and complications for both the mother and the developing fetus. Through personalized management strategies, healthcare providers can minimize these risks by selecting interventions that are tailored to the individual's medical history, gestational age, and underlying health conditions.

Enhanced Patient Engagement:

Personalized management empowers expectant mothers to actively participate in their healthcare decisions, fostering a sense of autonomy, ownership, and empowerment. By engaging patients as partners in the treatment process, healthcare providers can promote adherence to recommended interventions and improve patient outcomes.

Optimization of Resources:

In an era of constrained healthcare resources, personalized management strategies offer a cost-effective approach to pregnancy sickness management by minimizing unnecessary interventions, reducing healthcare utilization, and optimizing the allocation of resources towards interventions that yield the greatest benefit for patients.

Promotion of Holistic Well-being:

Pregnancy sickness extends beyond the realm of physical symptoms, encompassing a range of psychosocial and emotional challenges that can impact maternal well-being. Through personalized management, healthcare providers can address the holistic needs of expectant mothers, integrating psychosocial support, nutritional counseling, and complementary therapies into the treatment plan.

Long-term Health Outcomes: The management of pregnancy sickness has implications that extend beyond the duration of gestation, influencing maternal health outcomes and the well-being of the newborn. By adopting personalized management strategies, healthcare providers can mitigate the long-term effects of pregnancy sickness on maternal health, fostering optimal outcomes for both mother and child.

Introduction to Artificial Intelligence in Healthcare

In recent years, the integration of artificial intelligence (AI) into healthcare has heralded a new era of innovation, transformation, and promise. From diagnostic imaging to clinical decision support, AI technologies are revolutionizing the landscape of healthcare delivery, offering unprecedented opportunities to enhance patient outcomes, improve efficiency, and advance medical research.

15

In this section of "Utilizing Artificial Intelligence for Personalized Management of Pregnancy Sickness: Challenges, Opportunities, and Future Directions," we embark on a journey to explore the transformative potential of AI in reshaping maternal healthcare, with a specific focus on the management of pregnancy sickness.

Evolution of AI in Healthcare: The integration of AI into healthcare represents the culmination of decades of technological advancements, scientific discovery, and interdisciplinary collaboration. From the pioneering work of early researchers to the development of sophisticated machine learning algorithms, the evolution of AI has catalyzed a paradigm shift in the way healthcare is delivered, managed, and optimized.

Applications of AI in Healthcare: AI technologies encompass a diverse array of applications and functionalities, ranging from predictive analytics and natural language processing to computer vision and robotics. In the context of maternal healthcare, AI holds immense potential to revolutionize prenatal care, childbirth management, and postpartum support,

16

offering innovative solutions to address the unique needs and challenges faced by expectant mothers.

Clinical Decision Support Systems:

One of the most promising applications of AI in healthcare is the development of clinical decision support systems (CDSS), which leverage machine learning algorithms to analyze vast amounts of patient data, generate diagnostic insights, and inform evidence-based treatment recommendations. By providing healthcare providers with real-time access to actionable information, CDSS empower clinicians to make informed decisions, optimize treatment protocols, and improve patient outcomes.

Predictive Analytics and Risk Stratification:

AI-driven predictive analytics offer the ability to identify patterns, trends, and risk factors associated with pregnancy sickness, enabling early detection, intervention, and risk stratification. By analyzing a multitude of clinical variables, genetic markers, and environmental factors, predictive models can help healthcare providers anticipate and mitigate the onset and progression of pregnancy sickness, enhancing maternal and fetal well-being.

Personalized Medicine and Precision Healthcare:

At the heart of AI-driven healthcare is the concept of personalized medicine, which seeks to tailor medical interventions to the individual characteristics, preferences, and needs of each patient. Through the integration of genomic data, physiological parameters, and lifestyle factors, AI algorithms can develop personalized treatment plans that optimize therapeutic efficacy, minimize adverse effects, and promote patient-centered care.

Ethical and Regulatory Considerations:

As AI technologies continue to proliferate within the healthcare ecosystem, it is imperative to address the ethical, legal, and regulatory implications associated with their deployment. From concerns regarding data privacy and patient consent to issues of algorithmic bias and accountability, the ethical dimensions of AI in healthcare demand careful consideration and proactive mitigation strategies.

CHAPTER 1

UNDERSTANDING PREGNANCY SICKNESS

Pregnancy sickness, often colloquially referred to as morning sickness, represents a complex and multifaceted phenomenon that manifests in various forms and degrees of severity across expectant mothers. In this section of "Utilizing Artificial Intelligence for Personalized Management of Pregnancy Sickness: Challenges, Opportunities, and Future Directions," we embark on a journey to unravel the intricate nuances of pregnancy sickness, exploring its definition, prevalence, impact, and underlying mechanisms.

Definition and Clinical Presentation:

Pregnancy sickness encompasses a spectrum of symptoms, including nausea, vomiting, aversions to certain foods or smells, and general discomfort, which typically manifest during the early stages of pregnancy. While the term "morning sickness" suggests a temporal association with the morning hours, pregnancy sickness can occur at any time of the day or night, often persisting beyond the first trimester.

Prevalence and Variability:

Pregnancy sickness is a ubiquitous phenomenon, affecting approximately 70-80% of expectant mothers to varying degrees of severity. While the majority of cases are mild and self-limiting, a subset of individuals may experience more severe symptoms, leading to significant impairment of daily functioning and quality of life. The prevalence and severity of pregnancy sickness can be influenced by factors such as maternal age, parity, gestational age, and hormonal fluctuations.

Impact on Maternal Health and Well-being:

Beyond its physical manifestations, pregnancy sickness can exert a profound impact on the emotional, social, and psychological well-being of expectant mothers. Persistent nausea and vomiting can disrupt daily activities, impair occupational performance, and contribute to feelings of anxiety, depression, and isolation. Moreover, severe cases of pregnancy sickness, such as hyperemesis gravidarum, may necessitate hospitalization and intensive medical management to prevent dehydration, electrolyte imbalances, and maternal complications.

Underlying Mechanisms and Etiology:

The exact etiology of pregnancy sickness remains incompletely understood, although it is believed to involve a complex interplay of hormonal, physiological, genetic, and environmental factors. Fluctuations in hormone levels, particularly human chorionic gonadotropin (hCG) and estrogen, have been implicated in the pathogenesis of pregnancy sickness, although the precise mechanisms underlying symptom generation and maintenance remain subject to ongoing investigation.

Triggers and Risk Factors:

Pregnancy sickness can be triggered or exacerbated by a variety of factors, including certain foods, odors, visual stimuli, stress, fatigue, and gastrointestinal disturbances. Women with a history of motion sickness, migraines, or gastrointestinal disorders may be at increased risk of experiencing more severe symptoms during pregnancy. Additionally, genetic predispositions and familial patterns of pregnancy sickness suggest a hereditary component to the condition, although specific genetic markers have yet to be conclusively identified.

Management Strategies:

The management of pregnancy sickness typically involves a multimodal approach aimed at alleviating symptoms, minimizing complications, and optimizing maternal-fetal health outcomes. Dietary modifications, lifestyle interventions, pharmacological therapies, and complementary modalities such as acupuncture and acupressure may be employed based on the severity of symptoms and individual patient preferences.

As we deepen our understanding of pregnancy sickness and its myriad complexities, we lay the foundation for the development of innovative and personalized management strategies that harness the transformative potential of artificial intelligence. In the chapters that follow, we explore the integration of AI-driven decision support systems, predictive analytics, and personalized medicine approaches to optimize maternal health outcomes and revolutionize the standard of care for expectant mothers facing the challenges of pregnancy

Definition and Symptoms

Pregnancy sickness, also known as morning sickness, refers to a common physiological phenomenon experienced by many expectant mothers during pregnancy. In this section of "Utilizing Artificial Intelligence for Personalized Management of Pregnancy Sickness: Challenges, Opportunities, and Future Directions," we provide a comprehensive overview of the definition and symptoms associated with pregnancy sickness.

Definition: Pregnancy sickness encompasses a range of symptoms, including nausea, vomiting, aversions to certain foods or smells, and general discomfort, which typically manifest during the early stages of pregnancy. While the term "morning sickness" implies a temporal association with the morning hours, pregnancy sickness can occur at any time of the day or night, often persisting beyond the first trimester. It is important to note that pregnancy sickness varies in severity and duration among expectant mothers, with some individuals experiencing mild and self-limiting symptoms, while others may endure more severe manifestations requiring medical intervention.

Symptoms:

Nausea: Nausea is one of the hallmark symptoms of pregnancy sickness and is characterized by a sensation of queasiness or discomfort in the stomach, often accompanied by a desire to vomit. Nausea may be triggered or exacerbated by certain foods, odors, visual stimuli, stress, fatigue, or gastrointestinal disturbances.

Vomiting: Vomiting is another common symptom of pregnancy sickness, characterized by the forceful expulsion of stomach contents through the mouth. While vomiting is often preceded by feelings of nausea, it can occur suddenly and unpredictably, leading to feelings of discomfort and distress in affected individuals.

Food Aversions: Many expectant mothers experience aversions to certain foods or smells during pregnancy, particularly those that are strong-smelling, spicy, or fatty. Food aversions may contribute to dietary changes and preferences during pregnancy, as individuals seek to avoid triggering or exacerbating symptoms of pregnancy sickness.

Sensitivity to Odors: Pregnancy sickness may also be associated with heightened sensitivity to odors, with affected individuals experiencing aversion or discomfort in response to certain smells that they may have previously found tolerable or pleasant.

Fatigue and Discomfort: Pregnancy sickness can contribute to feelings of fatigue, lethargy, and general discomfort, which may impact daily activities, occupational performance, and quality of life for expectant mothers.

Severity and Duration: The severity and duration of pregnancy sickness can vary widely among individuals, with some experiencing mild and transient symptoms that resolve spontaneously, while others may endure more severe manifestations requiring medical management and intervention.

Prevalence and Impact on Pregnant Individuals

In this section of "Utilizing Artificial Intelligence for Personalized Management of Pregnancy Sickness: Challenges, Opportunities, and Future Directions," we delve into the prevalence and profound impact of pregnancy sickness on expectant mothers, highlighting the significance of understanding and addressing this common yet often underestimated condition.

Prevalence: Pregnancy sickness, encompassing symptoms such as nausea, vomiting, food aversions, and sensitivity to odors, affects a significant proportion of pregnant individuals worldwide. Studies estimate that approximately 70-80% of expectant mothers experience some degree of pregnancy sickness during the early stages of gestation, with the onset typically occurring within the first trimester. While the majority of cases are mild and self-limiting, a subset of individuals may experience more severe symptoms requiring medical intervention and support.

Impact on Pregnant Individuals:

The impact of pregnancy sickness extends beyond the realm of physical discomfort, exerting profound effects on the emotional, social, and psychological well-being of expectant mothers. For many individuals, persistent nausea and vomiting disrupt daily activities, impair occupational performance, and contribute to feelings of anxiety, depression, and isolation. The unpredictability and unpredictability of symptoms may lead to increased stress and uncertainty, further exacerbating the emotional toll of pregnancy sickness.

Moreover, severe cases of pregnancy sickness, such as hyperemesis gravidarum, can result in significant complications requiring hospitalization, intravenous hydration, and medical management to prevent dehydration, electrolyte imbalances, and maternal complications. The impact of pregnancy sickness extends beyond the individual level, affecting familial dynamics, social relationships, and maternal-infant bonding, thus underscoring the importance of early detection, intervention, and support.

Furthermore, pregnancy sickness may influence maternal health behaviors and pregnancy outcomes, including maternal weight gain, fetal growth, and neonatal outcomes. Individuals experiencing severe symptoms of pregnancy sickness may be at increased risk of nutritional deficiencies, dehydration, and adverse pregnancy outcomes, highlighting the importance of proactive management and multidisciplinary care.

By illuminating the prevalence and impact of pregnancy sickness on expectant mothers, we underscore the significance of developing personalized management strategies that address the unique needs and preferences of each individual. Through the integration of artificial intelligence, predictive analytics, and personalized medicine approaches, we aspire to redefine the standard of care for pregnancy sickness, optimizing maternal health outcomes and enhancing the well-being of expectant mothers and their families.

Current Approaches to Management

In this section of "Utilizing Artificial Intelligence for Personalized Management of Pregnancy Sickness: Challenges, Opportunities, and Future Directions," we explore the current approaches to managing pregnancy sickness, encompassing a range of interventions aimed at alleviating symptoms, minimizing complications, and optimizing maternal-fetal health outcomes.

Dietary Modifications: Dietary modifications represent a cornerstone of pregnancy sickness management, with recommendations focused on consuming small, frequent meals rich in complex carbohydrates and protein, while avoiding spicy, fatty, and strongly flavored foods that may exacerbate symptoms. Additionally, individuals are advised to stay hydrated by drinking fluids between meals and opting for bland, easily digestible snacks such as crackers or toast.

Lifestyle Interventions: Lifestyle interventions play a pivotal role in managing pregnancy sickness, with emphasis placed on implementing strategies to reduce stress, promote relaxation, and enhance overall well-being. Techniques such as mindfulness, deep breathing exercises, and progressive muscle relaxation may help alleviate symptoms of nausea and discomfort, while promoting a sense of calm and control.

Pharmacological Therapies:

Pharmacological therapies may be considered for individuals experiencing severe or persistent symptoms of pregnancy sickness, particularly those at risk of dehydration, electrolyte imbalances, or nutritional deficiencies. Antiemetic medications such as pyridoxine (vitamin B6) and doxylamine, as well as prescription medications like ondansetron, may be prescribed under the guidance of a healthcare provider to alleviate nausea and vomiting and improve maternal comfort and quality of life.

Complementary and Alternative Modalities:

Complementary and alternative modalities offer additional avenues for managing pregnancy sickness, with approaches ranging from acupuncture and acupressure to aromatherapy and herbal remedies. While evidence regarding the efficacy of these interventions remains limited, some individuals may find relief from symptoms through non-pharmacological means, particularly when integrated into a holistic and multidisciplinary treatment approach.

Supportive Care and Counseling:

Supportive care and counseling play an integral role in pregnancy sickness management, providing individuals with emotional support, practical guidance, and reassurance throughout the duration of gestation. Healthcare providers may offer counseling on coping strategies, stress management techniques, and communication strategies for navigating challenges related to pregnancy sickness within the context of familial, social, and occupational domains.

Multidisciplinary Collaboration:

Multidisciplinary collaboration among healthcare providers, including obstetricians, midwives, nurses, dietitians, and mental health professionals, is essential for ensuring comprehensive and coordinated care for individuals experiencing pregnancy sickness. By adopting a collaborative approach to management, healthcare teams can tailor interventions to address the unique needs and preferences of each individual, while optimizing maternal and fetal health outcomes.

CHAPTER 2
THE ROLE OF ARTIFICIAL INTELLIGENCE IN HEALTHCARE

In this pivotal section of "Utilizing Artificial Intelligence for Personalized Management of Pregnancy Sickness: Challenges, Opportunities, and Future Directions," we delve into the transformative role of artificial intelligence (AI) in revolutionizing healthcare delivery, particularly in the context of managing pregnancy sickness. By harnessing the power of AI-driven technologies, we aspire to enhance the quality of care, optimize treatment outcomes, and empower expectant mothers with personalized management strategies tailored to their unique needs and preferences.

Data Analytics and Pattern Recognition: At the heart of AI-driven healthcare lies the capacity to analyze vast quantities of data, extract meaningful insights, and identify patterns and trends that elude conventional methodologies. In the context of pregnancy sickness management, AI algorithms can leverage clinical data, genetic markers, physiological parameters, and environmental factors to discern patterns associated with symptom onset, severity, and response to treatment. By uncovering hidden correlations and predictive markers, AI enables healthcare providers to anticipate and preemptively address the needs of expectant mothers, optimizing maternal-fetal health outcomes and enhancing patient satisfaction.

Predictive Modeling and Risk Stratification:

AI-driven predictive modeling offers the potential to identify individuals at heightened risk of developing pregnancy sickness, enabling early intervention and targeted support initiatives. By integrating diverse datasets and machine learning algorithms, predictive models can stratify patients based on their risk profiles, guiding healthcare providers in allocating resources, prioritizing interventions, and tailoring treatment plans to address the specific needs of high-risk individuals. Moreover, predictive modeling facilitates the identification of modifiable risk factors and the development of preventive strategies aimed at mitigating the onset and progression of pregnancy sickness, fostering proactive and patient-centered care approaches.

Decision Support Systems and Personalized Medicine:

AI-driven decision support systems empower healthcare providers with real-time access to evidence-based guidelines, clinical pathways, and treatment recommendations, facilitating informed decision-making and personalized medicine approaches. By integrating patient-specific data, including medical history, demographic characteristics, and genetic predispositions, decision support systems enable clinicians to tailor interventions to the unique needs and preferences of each individual, optimizing therapeutic efficacy and minimizing adverse effects. Furthermore, AI algorithms can adapt and evolve in response to real-world feedback and clinical outcomes, refining treatment algorithms and enhancing the precision and effectiveness of personalized management strategies over time.

Ethical and Regulatory Considerations: As we harness the potential of AI in healthcare, it is imperative to address the ethical, legal, and regulatory considerations inherent in the deployment of these technologies. From concerns regarding data privacy and security to issues of algorithmic transparency and accountability, the ethical dimensions of AI demand careful consideration and proactive mitigation strategies. By fostering interdisciplinary collaborations, engaging stakeholders, and adhering to established ethical frameworks, we can ensure the responsible and equitable integration of AI-driven technologies into pregnancy sickness management, safeguarding patient rights, autonomy, and well-being.

Evolution and Advancements in AI Technologies

In this pivotal section of "Utilizing Artificial Intelligence for Personalized Management of Pregnancy Sickness: Challenges, Opportunities, and Future Directions," we embark on a journey to explore the remarkable evolution and advancements in artificial intelligence (AI) technologies that have reshaped the landscape of healthcare delivery, transforming the way we understand, diagnose, and manage complex medical conditions such as pregnancy sickness.

Origins of Artificial Intelligence:

The roots of artificial intelligence can be traced back to the pioneering work of early researchers and visionaries who sought to emulate human cognitive processes and reasoning capabilities using computational algorithms and models. From the seminal contributions of Alan Turing and John McCarthy to the development of expert systems and neural networks, the evolution of AI has been marked by continuous innovation, experimentation, and interdisciplinary collaboration across fields such as computer science, mathematics, neuroscience, and cognitive psychology.

Machine Learning and Deep Learning:

Central to the advancement of AI technologies is the paradigm of machine learning, which enables computers to learn from data, identify patterns, and make predictions without explicit programming.

Within the realm of healthcare, machine learning algorithms have revolutionized diagnostic imaging, predictive analytics, and clinical decision support, offering unprecedented insights into disease pathology, treatment response, and patient outcomes. Deep learning, a subset of machine learning characterized by hierarchical neural networks, has further enhanced the capabilities of AI systems, enabling the analysis of complex, high-dimensional datasets and the extraction of actionable insights from unstructured data sources such as medical images, electronic health records, and genomic sequences.

Natural Language Processing and Conversational AI:

Natural language processing (NLP) represents another frontier of AI innovation, enabling computers to understand, interpret, and generate human language in a manner that is contextually meaningful and semantically rich. In healthcare, NLP algorithms facilitate the extraction of clinical information from free-text documents, patient narratives, and medical literature, empowering healthcare providers with actionable insights and facilitating seamless communication between clinicians, patients, and other stakeholders. Conversational AI, powered by NLP and machine learning, has further revolutionized the delivery of healthcare services, enabling virtual assistants, chatbots, and voice-enabled interfaces to engage with patients, triage symptoms, and deliver personalized health information in real-time.

Explainable AI and Ethical Considerations:

As AI technologies continue to proliferate within the healthcare ecosystem, it is imperative to address the ethical, legal, and social implications associated with their deployment. From concerns regarding algorithmic bias and discrimination to issues of data privacy and transparency, the ethical dimensions of AI demand careful consideration and proactive mitigation strategies. Explainable AI, an emerging field focused on enhancing the transparency, interpretability, and accountability of AI systems, offers promising avenues for addressing these challenges and fostering trust, equity, and inclusivity within the healthcare domain.

Applications of AI in Healthcare

In this critical section of "Utilizing Artificial Intelligence for Personalized Management of Pregnancy Sickness: Challenges, Opportunities, and Future Directions," we delve into the diverse applications of artificial intelligence (AI) that have revolutionized healthcare delivery, offering innovative solutions to the challenges posed by pregnancy sickness and other complex medical conditions.

Diagnostic Imaging:

AI-driven algorithms have transformed the field of diagnostic imaging, enabling more accurate and efficient interpretation of medical images such as ultrasounds, MRIs, and CT scans. Machine learning algorithms can analyze vast datasets of radiological images, detect subtle abnormalities, and assist radiologists in identifying patterns indicative of pregnancy complications or other underlying conditions. By enhancing diagnostic accuracy and reducing interpretation times, AI-powered imaging solutions improve patient outcomes and streamline clinical workflows in prenatal care.

Clinical Decision Support:

AI-driven clinical decision support systems (CDSS) empower healthcare providers with real-time access to evidence-based guidelines, treatment protocols, and predictive analytics, enabling informed decision-making and personalized medicine approaches. In the context of pregnancy sickness management, CDSS algorithms can analyze patient data, assess risk factors, and recommend tailored interventions based on individualized risk profiles and treatment preferences. By integrating patient-specific information and clinical guidelines, CDSS facilitate proactive management strategies and optimize maternal-fetal health outcomes.

Predictive Analytics and Risk Stratification:

Predictive analytics leverage AI algorithms to identify patterns, trends, and risk factors associated with pregnancy sickness and other maternal health conditions. By analyzing diverse datasets encompassing clinical variables, genetic markers, and environmental factors, predictive models can stratify patients based on their risk profiles, anticipate adverse outcomes, and guide preventive interventions. Through early identification and risk stratification, predictive analytics enable healthcare providers to implement targeted interventions, optimize resource allocation, and mitigate the onset and progression of pregnancy complications.

Personalized Medicine and Treatment Optimization:

AI-driven approaches to personalized medicine leverage patient-specific data, including genomic information, physiological parameters, and lifestyle factors, to tailor interventions to the unique needs and preferences of each individual. In the context of pregnancy sickness management, personalized medicine approaches enable healthcare providers to develop customized treatment plans that optimize therapeutic efficacy, minimize adverse effects, and promote patient-centered care. By integrating clinical data with predictive modeling and decision support systems, personalized medicine algorithms facilitate precision healthcare delivery and enhance patient outcomes.

Natural Language Processing and Patient Engagement: Natural language processing (NLP) technologies enable computers to understand, interpret, and generate human language, facilitating seamless communication between healthcare providers and patients. In maternal healthcare, NLP-powered applications empower expectant mothers to access personalized health information, engage in informed decision-making, and communicate with healthcare providers through virtual assistants, chatbots, and voice-enabled interfaces. By promoting patient engagement and self-management, NLP technologies enhance the quality of care and foster collaborative partnerships between patients and providers.

Potential Benefits of AI in Pregnancy Sickness Management

In this pivotal section of "Utilizing Artificial Intelligence for Personalized Management of Pregnancy Sickness: Challenges,

Opportunities, and Future Directions," we explore the potential benefits of harnessing artificial intelligence (AI) technologies to optimize the management of pregnancy sickness, offering innovative solutions to enhance maternal health outcomes and improve the quality of care for expectant mothers.

Early Detection and Risk Assessment:

AI-driven predictive analytics enable early detection and risk assessment of pregnancy sickness, allowing healthcare providers to identify individuals at heightened risk of developing severe symptoms or complications. By analyzing diverse datasets encompassing clinical variables, genetic markers, and environmental factors, predictive models can stratify patients based on their risk profiles and facilitate targeted interventions to mitigate the onset and progression of pregnancy sickness.

Personalized Treatment Approaches:

AI-powered decision support systems enable personalized treatment approaches tailored to the unique needs and preferences of each individual. By integrating patient-specific data, including medical history, demographic characteristics, and symptom profiles, decision support algorithms can recommend tailored interventions, optimize therapeutic efficacy, and minimize adverse effects. Personalized treatment approaches empower expectant mothers to actively participate in their healthcare decisions, fostering a sense of autonomy, ownership, and empowerment throughout the management process.

Enhanced Clinical Decision-Making:

AI-driven clinical decision support systems empower healthcare providers with real-time access to evidence-based guidelines, treatment protocols, and predictive analytics, facilitating informed decision-making and optimizing patient outcomes. By integrating patient data, clinical guidelines, and best practices, decision support algorithms enable clinicians to navigate complex diagnostic and treatment dilemmas, streamline clinical workflows, and improve the efficiency and effectiveness of prenatal care delivery.

Improved Patient Engagement and Education: AI-powered patient engagement platforms facilitate communication, education, and support for expectant mothers throughout the pregnancy sickness management process. Virtual assistants, chatbots, and mobile applications empower patients to access personalized health information, track symptoms, and communicate with healthcare providers in real-time. By promoting patient engagement and self-management, AI-driven patient engagement platforms enhance adherence to treatment regimens, foster shared decision-making, and improve patient satisfaction and outcomes.

Data-driven Research and Innovation: AI technologies enable data-driven research and innovation in pregnancy sickness management, facilitating the discovery of novel biomarkers, therapeutic targets, and treatment modalities. By analyzing large-scale datasets encompassing clinical trials, electronic health records, and genomic sequences, AI algorithms can uncover hidden correlations, identify predictive markers, and inform the development of innovative interventions. Data-driven research powered by AI accelerates the pace of scientific discovery, fosters collaboration across disciplines, and drives positive change in maternal healthcare delivery.

CHAPTER 3

CHALLENGES IN PREGNANCY SICKNESS MANAGEMENT

In this critical section of "Utilizing Artificial Intelligence for Personalized Management of Pregnancy Sickness: Challenges, Opportunities, and Future Directions," we confront the multifaceted challenges that hinder effective management of pregnancy sickness, highlighting the complexities and limitations that must be addressed to optimize maternal health outcomes and enhance patient-centered care.

Heterogeneity of Symptoms:

Pregnancy sickness manifests as a spectrum of symptoms with varying degrees of severity and duration among expectant mothers. The heterogeneous nature of symptoms presents a challenge for healthcare providers in tailoring interventions to meet the diverse needs and preferences of each individual. Addressing the heterogeneity of symptoms requires personalized management strategies that leverage the transformative potential of artificial intelligence to accommodate the unique characteristics and experiences of each patient.

Limited Understanding of Etiology:

The exact etiology of pregnancy sickness remains incompletely understood, with factors such as hormonal fluctuations, genetic predispositions, and environmental triggers implicated in its pathogenesis. The lack of a comprehensive understanding of the underlying mechanisms hinders the development of targeted interventions and preventive strategies. Advancing our understanding of the etiology of pregnancy sickness requires interdisciplinary research efforts that integrate basic science, clinical investigation, and data-driven approaches to elucidate the complex interplay of factors contributing to symptom generation and maintenance.

Diagnostic Challenges:

Diagnosing pregnancy sickness can be challenging due to the overlap of symptoms with other medical conditions, such as gastroenteritis, migraines, and psychological disorders. The absence of objective biomarkers and standardized diagnostic criteria further complicates the diagnostic process, leading to delays in recognition and treatment initiation. Improving diagnostic accuracy and early detection of pregnancy sickness necessitates the development of sensitive and specific diagnostic tools, as well as the integration of clinical assessment, laboratory testing, and advanced imaging modalities into diagnostic algorithms.

Treatment Selection and Adherence:

The selection of optimal treatment modalities for pregnancy sickness is hindered by the lack of consensus regarding the efficacy and safety of available interventions. Pharmacological therapies, dietary modifications, and complementary modalities may yield variable responses among individuals, necessitating a personalized approach to treatment selection and monitoring. Additionally, poor adherence to treatment regimens poses a challenge for expectant mothers, particularly in the context of medication side effects, dietary restrictions, and

51

lifestyle modifications. Enhancing treatment adherence requires patient education, counseling, and ongoing support from healthcare providers to empower individuals to actively participate in their healthcare decisions and adhere to recommended interventions.

Ethical and Legal Considerations:

The integration of artificial intelligence into pregnancy sickness management raises ethical, legal, and social considerations related to data privacy, informed consent, algorithmic bias, and accountability. Safeguarding patient rights, autonomy, and confidentiality is paramount in the development and deployment of AI-driven technologies, requiring adherence to established ethical frameworks and regulatory standards. Additionally, addressing issues of algorithmic bias and transparency is essential to ensure equitable access to healthcare services and mitigate the risk of unintended consequences associated with algorithmic decision-making.

Variability in Symptoms and Triggers

In this critical section of "Utilizing Artificial Intelligence for Personalized Management of Pregnancy Sickness: Challenges, Opportunities, and Future Directions," we explore the diverse variability in symptoms and triggers associated with pregnancy sickness, highlighting the complexities and nuances that underscore the individualized nature of this common yet often challenging condition.

Symptom Variability:

Pregnancy sickness encompasses a wide spectrum of symptoms that can vary significantly among expectant mothers, both in terms of severity and duration. While nausea and vomiting are hallmark features of pregnancy sickness, the presentation and intensity of these symptoms can differ widely among individuals. Some women may experience mild, occasional nausea, while others may endure persistent, debilitating vomiting that necessitates medical intervention. Additionally, symptoms may fluctuate throughout the course of pregnancy, with periods of remission followed by exacerbations, further complicating management and treatment strategies.

Triggers of Symptoms:

The triggers of pregnancy sickness are multifactorial and can vary from one individual to another. While certain factors, such as hormonal fluctuations and changes in gastric motility, are implicated in the pathogenesis of pregnancy sickness, triggers can also include environmental stimuli, dietary factors, stress, fatigue, and psychological stressors. Common triggers may include strong odors, spicy or fatty foods, visual stimuli, and emotional stressors, although individual responses to these triggers can vary widely. Identifying and mitigating triggers of pregnancy sickness is essential for personalized management strategies that aim to minimize symptom severity and optimize maternal comfort and well-being.

Hormonal Influences:

Hormonal fluctuations, particularly changes in levels of human chorionic gonadotropin (hCG) and estrogen, are believed to play a central role in the pathophysiology of pregnancy sickness. While the exact mechanisms

54

underlying hormonal influences on symptom generation remain incompletely understood, research suggests that hCG may act on the central nervous system and gastrointestinal tract to induce nausea and vomiting. Additionally, fluctuations in estrogen levels may contribute to alterations in gastric motility and sensitivity, further exacerbating symptoms of pregnancy sickness. Understanding the hormonal influences on symptom variability is essential for developing targeted interventions and personalized management strategies that address the underlying pathophysiology of pregnancy sickness.

Individual Susceptibility and Genetic Predisposition:

Individual susceptibility to pregnancy sickness and its triggers is influenced by a variety of factors, including genetic predisposition, maternal age, parity, and pre-existing medical conditions. Women with a family history of pregnancy sickness or a personal history of motion sickness, migraines, or gastrointestinal disorders may be at increased risk of experiencing more severe symptoms during pregnancy. Additionally, genetic studies have identified potential candidate genes associated with pregnancy sickness, although the precise genetic mechanisms remain poorly understood. Further research is needed to elucidate the genetic determinants of pregnancy sickness and their implications for personalized management and treatment approaches.

By elucidating the variability in symptoms and triggers of pregnancy sickness, we lay the foundation for personalized management strategies that acknowledge the unique characteristics and experiences of each individual. Leveraging the transformative potential of artificial intelligence, predictive analytics, and personalized medicine approaches, we aspire to optimize maternal health outcomes and enhance the quality of care for expectant mothers facing the challenges of pregnancy sickness.

Limited Understanding of Underlying Mechanisms

In this critical section of "Utilizing Artificial Intelligence for Personalized Management of Pregnancy Sickness: Challenges,

56

Opportunities, and Future Directions," we confront the challenge posed by the limited understanding of the underlying mechanisms that contribute to the pathogenesis of pregnancy sickness. Despite its prevalence and significant impact on maternal health and well-being, pregnancy sickness remains a complex and multifaceted condition characterized by a lack of clarity regarding its etiology and underlying pathophysiology.

Hormonal Factors:

Hormonal fluctuations, particularly changes in levels of human chorionic gonadotropin (hCG), estrogen, and progesterone, are believed to play a central role in the pathogenesis of pregnancy sickness. While elevated levels of hCG have been associated with increased severity of symptoms, the exact mechanisms by which hCG influences symptom generation remain incompletely understood. Similarly, estrogen and progesterone may exert modulatory effects on gastric motility, sensitivity, and neurotransmitter pathways implicated in nausea and vomiting, although the precise mechanisms underlying hormonal influences require further elucidation.

Neurotransmitter Dysregulation:

Neurotransmitter dysregulation within the central nervous system (CNS), particularly involving serotonin, dopamine, and histamine pathways, has been implicated in the pathophysiology of pregnancy sickness. Alterations in neurotransmitter levels and receptor sensitivity may contribute to abnormalities in gastrointestinal motility, visceral perception, and emetic reflexes, leading to the manifestation of symptoms such as nausea and vomiting. However, the precise interactions between neurotransmitter systems and their role in pregnancy sickness remain poorly understood, highlighting the need for further research to elucidate the neurobiological mechanisms underlying symptom generation.

Genetic and Environmental Factors:

Genetic predisposition and environmental triggers are thought to interact synergistically in the development of pregnancy sickness. Women with a family history of pregnancy sickness or a personal history of motion sickness, migraines, or gastrointestinal disorders

58

may be at increased risk of experiencing more severe symptoms during pregnancy, suggesting a genetic component to susceptibility. However, the identification of specific genetic markers and the elucidation of their functional significance in pregnancy sickness remain areas of active investigation. Furthermore, environmental factors such as dietary habits, stress, and psychosocial factors may modulate the severity and frequency of symptoms, although the precise mechanisms by which these factors exert their effects require further exploration.

Interdisciplinary Research Efforts:

Addressing the limited understanding of underlying mechanisms in pregnancy sickness requires interdisciplinary research efforts that integrate basic science, clinical investigation, and data-driven approaches. By leveraging advanced technologies such as genomic sequencing, neuroimaging, and computational modeling, researchers can elucidate the complex interactions between genetic, hormonal, and environmental factors contributing to symptom generation. Moreover, collaborative initiatives involving obstetricians, gastroenterologists, neuroscientists, and geneticists are essential for advancing our understanding of pregnancy sickness and translating research findings into innovative diagnostic and therapeutic strategies.

By acknowledging the challenges posed by the limited understanding of underlying mechanisms in pregnancy sickness, we underscore the importance of continued research efforts and interdisciplinary collaborations aimed at unraveling the complexities of this common yet enigmatic condition. Through the integration of artificial intelligence, predictive analytics, and personalized medicine approaches, we aspire to deepen our understanding of pregnancy sickness and develop targeted interventions that optimize maternal health outcomes and enhance patient-centered care.

Existing Treatment Limitations

In this crucial section of "Utilizing Artificial Intelligence for Personalized Management of Pregnancy Sickness: Challenges,

Opportunities, and Future Directions," we confront the existing limitations of treatment options available for pregnancy sickness. Despite advancements in medical science and clinical practice, the management of pregnancy sickness continues to present challenges, underscoring the need for innovative approaches to address the diverse needs and preferences of expectant mothers.

Limited Efficacy of Pharmacological Therapies:

Pharmacological therapies, including antiemetic medications such as pyridoxine (vitamin B6), doxylamine, and ondansetron, are commonly prescribed for the management of pregnancy sickness. While these medications can provide symptomatic relief for some individuals, their efficacy is variable, and many women may experience only partial or transient improvement in symptoms. Moreover, concerns regarding the safety of pharmacological interventions during pregnancy, particularly with respect to fetal development and teratogenicity, necessitate cautious consideration of the risks and benefits associated with medication use.

Challenges with Dietary Modifications:

Dietary modifications represent a cornerstone of pregnancy sickness management, with recommendations focused on consuming small, frequent meals and avoiding triggers such as spicy, fatty, and strongly flavored foods. However, adherence to dietary restrictions can be challenging for many expectant mothers, particularly in the context of food aversions and nausea-induced appetite suppression. Moreover, the effectiveness of dietary modifications may vary among individuals, and some women may find that certain dietary interventions provide limited relief from symptoms.

Limited Access to Supportive Care:

Access to supportive care and counseling services for pregnancy sickness management may be limited, particularly in underserved communities or rural areas where healthcare resources are scarce. Many expectant mothers may face barriers to accessing comprehensive prenatal care, including limited availability of specialized providers, financial constraints, and logistical challenges. As a result, some women may struggle to access the supportive care and counseling services needed to cope with the physical and emotional toll of pregnancy sickness, exacerbating feelings of isolation and distress.

Lack of Personalized Treatment Approaches:

The one-size-fits-all approach to pregnancy sickness management fails to account for the individual variability in symptoms, triggers, and treatment responses among expectant mothers. Current treatment modalities often lack personalization and may not adequately address the unique needs and preferences of each individual. Moreover, the limited understanding of the underlying mechanisms driving pregnancy sickness further complicates the development of personalized treatment approaches tailored to the specific characteristics and experiences of each patient.

Stigma and Misconceptions:

Stigma and misconceptions surrounding

pregnancy sickness may contribute to underreporting and undertreatment of symptoms among expectant mothers. Despite being a common and often debilitating condition, pregnancy sickness is sometimes trivialized or dismissed as a normal part of pregnancy, leading to delays in recognition and intervention. Furthermore, cultural and societal attitudes towards pregnancy sickness may vary, with some women feeling ashamed or embarrassed to seek help for their symptoms due to fear of judgment or stigma.

Addressing the existing limitations of treatment options for pregnancy sickness requires a multifaceted approach that integrates clinical expertise, patient-centered care principles, and innovative technologies such as artificial intelligence. By leveraging the transformative potential of AI-driven decision support systems, predictive analytics, and personalized medicine approaches, we aspire to redefine the standard of care for pregnancy sickness, optimize maternal health outcomes, and enhance the quality of life for expectant mothers and their families.

CHAPTER 4

LEVERAGING AI FOR PERSONALIZED MANAGEMENT

In this pivotal section of "Utilizing Artificial Intelligence for Personalized Management of Pregnancy Sickness: Challenges, Opportunities, and Future Directions," we explore the transformative potential of artificial intelligence (AI) in revolutionizing the management of pregnancy sickness, offering innovative solutions to address the diverse needs and preferences of expectant mothers through personalized care approaches.

Predictive Analytics and Risk Stratification: AI-driven predictive analytics empower healthcare providers with the ability to identify individuals at heightened risk of developing pregnancy sickness and its associated complications. By analyzing diverse datasets encompassing clinical variables, genetic markers, and environmental factors, predictive models can stratify patients

65

based on their risk profiles and guide targeted interventions tailored to the specific needs of each individual. Through early detection and risk stratification, predictive analytics enable proactive management strategies that optimize maternal-fetal health outcomes and enhance patient satisfaction.

Decision Support Systems for Treatment Optimization:

AI-powered decision support systems facilitate informed decision-making and personalized treatment optimization in pregnancy sickness management. By integrating patient-specific data, clinical guidelines, and best practices, decision support algorithms enable clinicians to tailor interventions to the unique characteristics and preferences of each patient, optimizing therapeutic efficacy and minimizing adverse effects. Moreover, decision support systems can adapt and evolve in response to real-time feedback and clinical outcomes, refining treatment algorithms and enhancing the precision and effectiveness of personalized management strategies over time.

Personalized Medicine Approaches: AI-driven personalized medicine approaches revolutionize the delivery of healthcare by leveraging patient-specific data, including genomic information, physiological parameters, and lifestyle factors, to tailor interventions to the unique needs of each individual. In the context of pregnancy sickness management, personalized medicine approaches enable healthcare providers to develop customized treatment plans that optimize therapeutic efficacy, minimize adverse effects, and promote patient-centered care. By integrating clinical data with predictive modeling and decision support systems, personalized medicine algorithms facilitate precision healthcare delivery and enhance patient outcomes.

Patient Engagement and Self-Management: AI-powered patient engagement platforms empower expectant mothers to actively participate in their healthcare decisions and self-management strategies. Through virtual assistants, chatbots, and mobile applications, patients can access personalized health information, track symptoms, and communicate with healthcare providers in real-time. By promoting patient engagement and self-management, AI-driven patient engagement platforms enhance adherence to treatment regimens, foster shared decision-making, and improve patient satisfaction and outcomes.

Ethical and Regulatory Considerations:

As we leverage AI for personalized management of pregnancy sickness, it is imperative to address the ethical, legal, and regulatory considerations inherent in the deployment of these technologies. From concerns regarding data privacy and security to issues of algorithmic transparency and accountability, the ethical dimensions of AI demand careful consideration and proactive mitigation strategies. By fostering interdisciplinary collaborations, engaging stakeholders, and adhering to established ethical frameworks, we can ensure the responsible and equitable integration of AI-driven technologies into pregnancy sickness management, safeguarding patient rights, autonomy, and well-being.

Data Analytics and Pattern Recognition

In this critical section of "Utilizing Artificial Intelligence for Personalized Management of Pregnancy Sickness: Challenges, Opportunities, and Future Directions," we delve into the transformative potential of data analytics and pattern recognition in revolutionizing the management of pregnancy sickness. By harnessing the power of artificial intelligence (AI) and advanced data analytics techniques, we aspire to uncover hidden insights, identify predictive patterns, and personalize treatment strategies tailored to the unique needs and preferences of expectant mothers.

Data Integration and Analysis:

Data integration lies at the heart of AI-driven approaches to pregnancy sickness management. By aggregating diverse datasets encompassing clinical variables, genetic markers, environmental factors, and patient-reported outcomes, healthcare providers can gain a comprehensive understanding of the complex interplay of factors contributing to symptom onset, severity, and progression. Advanced data analytics techniques, including machine learning algorithms and statistical modeling, enable clinicians to analyze large-scale datasets, identify meaningful patterns, and extract actionable insights that inform clinical decision-making and personalized treatment approaches.

Predictive Modeling and Risk Assessment:

Predictive modeling represents a powerful tool for identifying individuals at heightened risk of developing pregnancy sickness and its associated complications. By leveraging machine learning algorithms, predictive models can analyze historical patient data, identify predictive markers, and stratify patients based on their risk profiles. Through early detection and risk assessment, predictive modeling facilitates proactive management strategies that optimize maternal-fetal health outcomes, enhance patient satisfaction, and minimize healthcare costs associated with preventable complications.

Pattern Recognition and Treatment Optimization:

Pattern recognition algorithms enable healthcare

providers to identify common symptom clusters, treatment response patterns, and disease trajectories among expectant mothers with pregnancy sickness. By analyzing longitudinal patient data and identifying recurrent patterns, clinicians can tailor interventions to address the specific needs and preferences of each individual. Moreover, pattern recognition algorithms can adapt and evolve in response to real-world feedback and clinical outcomes, refining treatment algorithms and enhancing the precision and effectiveness of personalized management strategies over time.

Clinical Decision Support Systems:

Clinical decision support systems (CDSS) empower healthcare providers with real-time access to evidence-based guidelines, treatment protocols, and predictive analytics, facilitating informed decision-making and personalized medicine approaches. By integrating patient-specific data with clinical guidelines and best practices, CDSS algorithms enable clinicians to navigate complex diagnostic and treatment dilemmas, streamline clinical workflows, and improve the efficiency and effectiveness of prenatal care delivery. Moreover, CDSS can facilitate shared decision-making and collaborative care models that empower patients to actively participate in their healthcare decisions and treatment plans.

Development of AI-Driven Decision Support Systems

In this critical section of "Utilizing Artificial Intelligence for Personalized Management of Pregnancy Sickness: Challenges, Opportunities, and Future Directions," we explore the development and implementation of AI-driven decision support systems (DSS) in revolutionizing the management of pregnancy sickness. By harnessing the capabilities of artificial intelligence (AI), decision support systems empower healthcare providers with real-time access to evidence-based guidelines, treatment protocols, and predictive analytics, facilitating informed decision-making and personalized care approaches tailored to the unique needs and preferences of expectant mothers.

Integration of Patient Data:

AI-driven decision support systems integrate diverse sources of patient data, including clinical variables, genetic markers, environmental factors, and patient-reported outcomes, to generate comprehensive patient profiles that inform clinical decision-making. By aggregating and analyzing longitudinal patient data, decision support systems enable clinicians to identify trends, patterns, and risk factors associated with pregnancy sickness and its complications, facilitating proactive management strategies that optimize maternal-fetal health outcomes.

Machine Learning Algorithms:

Machine learning algorithms lie at the core of AI-driven decision support systems, enabling the analysis of large-scale datasets and the identification of meaningful patterns and associations. Supervised learning algorithms, such as logistic regression and random forest classifiers, can predict the likelihood of pregnancy sickness onset, severity, and progression based on historical patient data. Unsupervised learning algorithms, such as clustering and association rule mining, can identify common symptom clusters and treatment response patterns among expectant mothers, facilitating personalized treatment approaches tailored to individual needs.

Predictive Analytics for Risk Stratification:

Predictive analytics algorithms within decision support systems enable risk stratification of expectant mothers based on their likelihood of developing pregnancy sickness and its associated complications. By analyzing demographic characteristics, medical history, and clinical biomarkers, predictive models can identify individuals at heightened risk of adverse outcomes, facilitating early intervention and preventive strategies that optimize maternal and fetal health outcomes.

Real-Time Clinical Decision Support:

AI-driven decision support systems provide healthcare providers with real-time access to evidence-based guidelines, treatment protocols, and best practices for pregnancy sickness management. Through intuitive user interfaces and interoperable electronic health record systems, decision support systems deliver actionable insights and recommendations at the point of care, facilitating informed decision-making and enhancing the efficiency and effectiveness of prenatal care delivery.

Continuous Learning and Adaptation:

AI-driven decision support systems continuously learn and adapt in response to real-world feedback and clinical outcomes, refining treatment algorithms and enhancing the precision and effectiveness of personalized management strategies over time. By leveraging reinforcement learning and natural language processing techniques, decision support systems can extract knowledge from unstructured data sources such as medical literature, patient narratives, and expert opinions, further enhancing their decision-making capabilities and clinical utility.

Personalized Treatment Strategies

In this pivotal section of "Utilizing Artificial Intelligence for Personalized Management of Pregnancy Sickness: Challenges, Opportunities, and Future Directions," we explore the development and implementation of personalized treatment strategies for pregnancy sickness. By leveraging the capabilities of artificial intelligence (AI) and advanced data analytics techniques, personalized treatment approaches empower healthcare providers to tailor interventions to the unique needs, preferences, and characteristics of expectant mothers, optimizing maternal health outcomes and enhancing patient satisfaction.

Patient-Centered Care: Personalized treatment strategies prioritize patient-centered care principles, placing the individual needs and preferences of expectant mothers at the forefront of clinical decision-making. By engaging patients as active partners in their healthcare journey, healthcare providers foster collaborative relationships built on trust, empathy, and shared decision-making. Personalized treatment plans are co-created with patients, taking into account their values, beliefs, cultural backgrounds, and treatment goals, ensuring that interventions align with their preferences and priorities.

Comprehensive Patient Assessment: Personalized treatment strategies begin with a comprehensive assessment of each patient's medical history, demographic characteristics, genetic predispositions, and environmental exposures. Through detailed clinical evaluations, healthcare providers gain insights into the unique factors contributing to the onset, severity, and progression of pregnancy sickness in each individual. Advanced data analytics techniques, including machine learning algorithms and predictive modeling, enable clinicians to identify predictive markers and risk factors associated with adverse outcomes, guiding personalized treatment approaches tailored to individual needs.

Multimodal Interventions:

Personalized treatment strategies for pregnancy sickness encompass multimodal interventions that address the diverse array of symptoms, triggers, and contributing factors affecting expectant mothers. Pharmacological therapies, dietary modifications, complementary modalities, and lifestyle interventions may be combined in a holistic treatment approach that targets symptom relief, improves quality of life, and promotes maternal-fetal well-being. By tailoring interventions to address the specific needs and preferences of each individual, personalized treatment strategies optimize therapeutic efficacy, minimize adverse effects, and enhance patient satisfaction.

Adaptive Treatment Algorithms:

Personalized treatment strategies leverage adaptive treatment algorithms that evolve in response to real-time feedback and clinical outcomes, refining intervention plans and optimizing treatment regimens over time. Through continuous monitoring and assessment, healthcare providers adjust treatment parameters, dosage levels, and intervention modalities to accommodate changes in patient symptoms, preferences, and treatment responses. Artificial intelligence-driven decision support systems facilitate the dynamic adjustment of treatment algorithms, enabling personalized care delivery that adapts to the unique needs and circumstances of each patient.

Shared Decision-Making:

Personalized treatment strategies emphasize shared decision-making between healthcare providers and patients, empowering expectant mothers to actively participate in their healthcare decisions and treatment plans. Through open communication, education, and shared deliberation, patients are empowered to make informed choices regarding their care, weighing the risks, benefits, and alternatives of different treatment options. Healthcare providers serve as trusted guides and advocates, offering support, guidance, and reassurance throughout the decision-making process, fostering collaborative partnerships that promote patient autonomy and empowerment.

CHAPTER 5

ETHICAL AND PRIVACY CONSIDERATIONS

In this critical section of "Utilizing Artificial Intelligence for Personalized Management of Pregnancy Sickness: Challenges, Opportunities, and Future Directions," we address the ethical and privacy considerations inherent in the utilization of artificial intelligence (AI) for personalized management of pregnancy sickness. While AI-driven technologies offer unprecedented opportunities to improve maternal health outcomes and enhance patient-centered care, they also raise complex ethical and privacy concerns that must be carefully navigated to safeguard patient rights, autonomy, and confidentiality.

Data Privacy and Security: The collection, storage, and analysis of sensitive patient data pose significant privacy and security risks that must be addressed to protect patient confidentiality and mitigate the risk of unauthorized access or data breaches. Healthcare organizations must implement robust data encryption, access controls, and authentication mechanisms to safeguard patient information against cyber threats and malicious attacks. Additionally, adherence to established data protection regulations, such as the Health Insurance Portability and Accountability Act (HIPAA) in the United States, is essential to ensure compliance with legal and regulatory requirements governing patient privacy and data security.

Informed Consent and Transparency:

Informed consent is a cornerstone of ethical healthcare practice, requiring healthcare providers to fully disclose the risks, benefits, and alternatives of AI-driven interventions to patients, enabling them to make informed decisions regarding their care. Patients must be provided with clear and transparent information regarding the purposes, scope, and potential implications of AI-driven technologies, including the collection, use, and sharing of their health data for research and clinical purposes. Moreover, patients should have the opportunity to withdraw consent and exercise control over the use of their data, respecting their autonomy and right to privacy.

Algorithmic Bias and Fairness:

Algorithmic bias represents a significant ethical concern in the development and deployment of AI-driven technologies, leading to disparities in healthcare access, diagnosis, and treatment outcomes among diverse patient populations. Biases embedded within AI algorithms may perpetuate systemic inequalities and exacerbate existing disparities in healthcare delivery, particularly among marginalized and underserved communities. Healthcare providers must proactively identify and mitigate algorithmic biases through rigorous testing, validation, and ongoing monitoring of AI algorithms to ensure fairness, equity, and inclusivity in decision-making processes.

Accountability and Transparency:

Healthcare providers bear a responsibility to uphold ethical principles of accountability, transparency, and integrity in the development, deployment, and evaluation of AI-driven technologies. Transparent reporting of AI algorithms, methodologies, and decision-making processes is essential to foster trust and confidence among patients, healthcare providers, and regulatory authorities. Moreover, mechanisms for auditing, oversight, and accountability should be established to monitor the performance, accuracy, and ethical compliance of AI-driven systems, ensuring that they adhere to established ethical standards and regulatory guidelines.

Patient Empowerment and Advocacy:

Patient empowerment and advocacy play a crucial role in promoting ethical healthcare practices and ensuring that patient rights and interests are respected and protected. Patients should be empowered to actively participate in discussions regarding the ethical and privacy implications of AI-driven technologies, advocating for policies and practices that prioritize their autonomy, dignity, and well-being. Moreover, healthcare providers should engage in transparent communication and shared decision-making with patients, fostering collaborative partnerships built on mutual respect, trust, and empathy.

83

Protection of Patient Data

In this crucial section of "Utilizing Artificial Intelligence for Personalized Management of Pregnancy Sickness: Challenges, Opportunities, and Future Directions," we delve into the paramount importance of protecting patient data in the context of utilizing artificial intelligence (AI) for personalized management of pregnancy sickness. As AI-driven technologies increasingly permeate healthcare settings, ensuring the privacy, security, and confidentiality of patient information is imperative to maintain patient trust, uphold ethical standards, and comply with regulatory requirements.

Data Encryption and Access Controls:

Effective protection of patient data begins with robust data encryption and access controls to safeguard sensitive health information from unauthorized access, interception, or manipulation. Healthcare organizations must implement encryption protocols to secure data both at rest and in transit, mitigating the risk of data breaches and unauthorized disclosures. Access controls, including role-based permissions and multi-factor authentication mechanisms, restrict access to patient data to authorized personnel only, minimizing the potential for insider threats and unauthorized data access.

Secure Data Storage and Transmission:

Secure data storage and transmission mechanisms are essential to prevent data loss, corruption, or unauthorized disclosure throughout the data lifecycle. Healthcare providers must implement secure storage solutions, such as encrypted databases and cloud-based platforms with stringent access controls and audit trails, to protect patient data from cyber threats and data breaches. Similarly, secure transmission protocols, including secure sockets layer (SSL) encryption and virtual private networks (VPNs), ensure the confidentiality and integrity of data transmitted between healthcare systems, devices, and stakeholders.

Compliance with Regulatory Requirements:

Compliance with regulatory requirements, such as the Health Insurance Portability and

Accountability Act (HIPAA) in the United States and the General Data Protection Regulation (GDPR) in the European Union, is paramount to safeguard patient privacy and ensure legal and ethical standards in data handling practices. Healthcare organizations must adhere to established data protection regulations, including requirements for data minimization, purpose limitation, and data subject rights, to protect patient rights and mitigate the risk of regulatory sanctions or legal liabilities.

Data Anonymization and De-identification: Anonymization and de-identification techniques are employed to remove or obfuscate personally identifiable information (PII) from patient data, reducing the risk of re-identification and protecting patient privacy in research and analytics activities. Healthcare providers must implement robust anonymization protocols, including differential privacy techniques and data masking algorithms, to anonymize sensitive health information while preserving the utility and integrity of datasets for research and analysis purposes.

Ethical Use and Responsible Data Governance: Ethical use and responsible data governance practices are essential to ensure that patient data is utilized in a manner that respects patient autonomy, dignity, and rights. Healthcare organizations must establish clear policies and procedures governing the collection, use, and disclosure of patient data, including mechanisms for obtaining informed consent, transparent communication, and patient participation in decision-making processes. Moreover, healthcare providers should prioritize transparency, accountability, and stakeholder engagement in data governance initiatives, fostering trust and confidence among patients, healthcare providers, and regulatory authorities.

Informed Consent and Transparency

In this pivotal section of "Utilizing Artificial Intelligence for Personalized Management of Pregnancy Sickness: Challenges, Opportunities, and Future Directions," we delve into the fundamental principles of informed consent and transparency in the context of utilizing artificial intelligence (AI) for personalized management of pregnancy sickness. As AI-driven technologies play an increasingly prominent role in healthcare delivery, ensuring that patients are fully informed about the implications, risks, and benefits of AI applications is essential to uphold patient autonomy, foster trust, and promote ethical decision-making.

Patient-Centered Communication:

Effective communication lies at the heart of informed consent, empowering patients to make autonomous decisions regarding their healthcare. Healthcare providers must engage in patient-centered communication that fosters open dialogue, active listening, and shared decision-making, enabling patients to express their preferences, concerns, and values. Through clear and transparent communication, patients are provided with relevant information about the nature, purpose, and potential implications of AI-driven interventions, empowering them to make informed choices regarding their care.

Disclosure of Risks and Benefits:

Informed consent requires healthcare providers to disclose the potential risks, benefits, and uncertainties associated with AI-driven interventions, enabling patients to weigh the potential advantages and disadvantages of different treatment options. Patients should be informed about the limitations, biases, and uncertainties inherent in AI algorithms, including the potential for algorithmic errors, data biases, and unintended consequences. Moreover, patients should be educated about the potential benefits of AI applications, including improved diagnostic accuracy, personalized treatment approaches, and enhanced healthcare delivery.

Transparency in Data Use and Sharing:

Transparency in data use and sharing is essential to foster trust and accountability in the utilization of patient data for AI-driven applications. Healthcare providers must be transparent about the purposes, scope, and implications of data collection, processing, and sharing activities, including the types of data collected, the entities involved, and the safeguards implemented to protect patient privacy and confidentiality. Patients should be informed about their rights regarding data access, correction, and deletion, empowering them to exercise control over the use of their health information.

Consent for Research and Innovation:

Informed consent extends beyond clinical care to encompass research and innovation activities involving AI-driven technologies. Patients should be provided with clear and understandable information about the research objectives, methodologies, and potential risks and benefits of participating in research studies or clinical trials involving AI applications. Additionally, patients should be informed about their rights regarding data sharing, publication, and intellectual property, ensuring that their interests and contributions are respected and protected in research endeavors.

Ongoing Communication and Education:

Informed consent is an ongoing process that requires continuous communication and education to ensure that patients remain informed and engaged throughout the course of their healthcare journey. Healthcare providers should provide patients with opportunities to ask questions, seek clarification, and express their preferences regarding AI-driven interventions, fostering a collaborative partnership built on trust, respect, and shared decision-making. Moreover, patients should be empowered with access to reliable sources of information and educational resources that enhance their understanding of AI technologies and their implications for healthcare delivery.

Mitigating Bias and Algorithmic Fairness

In this critical section of "Utilizing Artificial Intelligence for Personalized Management of Pregnancy Sickness: Challenges, Opportunities, and Future Directions," we address the imperative need to mitigate bias and ensure algorithmic fairness in the utilization of artificial intelligence (AI) for personalized management of pregnancy sickness. As AI-driven technologies increasingly influence healthcare decision-making, it is paramount to identify and address biases that may perpetuate inequities, disparities, and injustices in healthcare delivery.

Awareness and Identification of Bias:

The first step in mitigating bias is to raise awareness and systematically identify potential sources of bias within AI algorithms and datasets. Healthcare providers must critically examine the data sources, sampling methodologies, and feature selection processes used to train AI models, identifying biases stemming from historical disparities, demographic imbalances, and societal prejudices. Through rigorous data auditing and algorithmic validation, healthcare organizations can uncover hidden biases and disparities that may compromise the fairness and equity of AI-driven interventions.

Bias Detection and Quantification:

Quantitative methods and metrics are employed to detect, measure, and quantify the extent of bias within AI algorithms and decision-making processes. Fairness metrics, such as disparate impact analysis, demographic parity, and equal opportunity metrics, enable healthcare providers to assess the fairness and equity of AI-driven interventions across diverse patient populations. Additionally, bias detection algorithms and model interpretability techniques help identify discriminatory patterns, feature biases, and decision-making disparities that may disproportionately impact marginalized or vulnerable patient groups.

Algorithmic Transparency and Explainability:

Algorithmic transparency and explainability are essential to enhance accountability, trust, and user comprehension of AI-driven decision-making processes. Healthcare providers must adopt transparent and interpretable AI algorithms that enable stakeholders to understand the underlying factors driving algorithmic decisions, including feature importance, decision rules, and model predictions. Through visualizations, explanations, and model documentation, healthcare organizations can promote algorithmic transparency and empower stakeholders to assess the fairness and ethical implications of AI-driven interventions.

93

Fairness-Aware Algorithm Design:

Fairness-aware algorithm design integrates principles of fairness, equity, and social justice into the development and deployment of AI-driven technologies. Healthcare providers must prioritize fairness-awareness in algorithm design, incorporating fairness constraints, regularization techniques, and fairness-aware optimization objectives to mitigate bias and promote algorithmic fairness. Moreover, interdisciplinary collaborations between data scientists, ethicists, and domain experts are essential to integrate diverse perspectives and ethical considerations into algorithmic decision-making processes.

Bias Mitigation Strategies:

Bias mitigation strategies encompass a spectrum of interventions aimed at reducing, mitigating, or eliminating biases within AI algorithms and decision-making processes. Proactive strategies, such as data preprocessing techniques, bias-aware sampling methodologies, and diversity-enhancing data augmentation, help mitigate biases at the data level, ensuring that training datasets reflect the diversity and representativeness of patient populations. Additionally, post-processing techniques, such as calibration, reweighting, and bias mitigation algorithms, enable healthcare providers to adjust algorithmic outputs and decision thresholds to promote fairness and equity in healthcare delivery.

CHAPTER 6

FUTURE DIRECTIONS AND RESEARCH OPPORTUNITIES

In this forward-looking section of "Utilizing Artificial Intelligence for Personalized Management of Pregnancy Sickness: Challenges, Opportunities, and Future Directions," we explore emerging trends, innovative approaches, and research opportunities shaping the future of AI-driven personalized management of pregnancy sickness. As the field of maternal healthcare continues to evolve, novel technologies, interdisciplinary collaborations, and research initiatives hold the potential to revolutionize prenatal care delivery, optimize maternal-fetal health outcomes, and enhance the quality of life for expectant mothers.

Integration of Multiomic Data:

Future research endeavors will focus on integrating multiomic data, including genomics, transcriptomics, proteomics, and metabolomics, to unravel the complex molecular mechanisms underlying pregnancy sickness and its associated complications. By leveraging advanced omics technologies and bioinformatics approaches, researchers can identify novel biomarkers, genetic variants, and molecular pathways associated with pregnancy sickness, guiding the development of targeted interventions and precision medicine approaches tailored to individual patient profiles.

Implementation of Wearable and Sensor Technologies:

The proliferation of wearable devices and sensor technologies presents unprecedented opportunities to monitor maternal health parameters, track symptom progression, and predict pregnancy-related complications in real-time. Future research initiatives will explore the integration of wearable sensors, smartphone applications, and remote monitoring platforms to collect continuous physiological data, behavioral insights, and environmental exposures, enabling early detection of pregnancy sickness and personalized intervention strategies.

Artificial Intelligence for Predictive Modeling: Advancements in artificial intelligence and machine learning algorithms will drive the development of predictive models capable of forecasting pregnancy sickness onset, severity, and progression with unprecedented accuracy and reliability. Future research efforts will focus on refining predictive analytics frameworks, enhancing model interpretability, and integrating multimodal data sources to improve risk stratification and inform personalized management strategies for expectant mothers.

Implementation of Virtual Health Platforms: Virtual health platforms, including telemedicine, virtual reality, and telemonitoring solutions, will play an increasingly prominent role in delivering personalized care to pregnant individuals, particularly in remote or underserved areas. Future research will explore the integration of virtual health technologies into prenatal care delivery models, enabling seamless access to healthcare services, remote consultations, and patient

education resources tailored to the unique needs and preferences of expectant mothers.

Ethical and Social Implications:

Future research endeavors will address the ethical, legal, and social implications of AI-driven personalized management of pregnancy sickness, including issues related to privacy, consent, equity, and algorithmic transparency. Interdisciplinary collaborations between healthcare providers, ethicists, policymakers, and community stakeholders will foster dialogue, consensus-building, and the development of ethical frameworks that promote patient-centered care, respect patient autonomy, and uphold principles of justice and fairness in healthcare delivery.

Longitudinal Studies and Clinical Trials:

Longitudinal studies and large-scale clinical trials will provide critical insights into the long-term effectiveness, safety, and patient outcomes associated with AI-driven personalized management strategies for pregnancy sickness. Future research initiatives will prioritize the design and implementation of prospective cohort studies, randomized controlled trials, and real-world evidence studies to evaluate the efficacy, cost-effectiveness, and patient satisfaction of AI-driven interventions in diverse clinical settings.

Emerging Technologies and Innovations

In this dynamic section of "Utilizing Artificial Intelligence for Personalized Management of Pregnancy Sickness: Challenges, Opportunities, and Future Directions," we delve into the cutting-edge technologies and innovative approaches that are reshaping the landscape of personalized management for pregnancy sickness. As the field of maternal healthcare continues to evolve, the integration of emerging technologies holds the potential to revolutionize prenatal care delivery, enhance patient outcomes, and improve the quality of life for expectant mothers.

Genomic Medicine and Precision Health: Genomic medicine and precision health initiatives are transforming our understanding of pregnancy sickness by

100

unraveling the genetic underpinnings and molecular mechanisms contributing to its onset and progression. Advances in next-generation sequencing technologies, genome-wide association studies, and computational genomics enable researchers to identify genetic variants, gene expression profiles, and biological pathways associated with pregnancy sickness susceptibility. By integrating genomic data into personalized management strategies, healthcare providers can tailor interventions and treatment approaches to individual genetic profiles, optimizing therapeutic efficacy and minimizing adverse effects.

Digital Health and Mobile Applications:

Digital health technologies, including mobile applications, wearable devices, and remote monitoring platforms, are empowering expectant mothers to actively participate in their healthcare management and monitor their health parameters in real-time. Mobile applications enable users to track symptoms, dietary intake, and medication adherence, providing valuable insights into symptom progression and treatment response. Wearable devices, such as smartwatches and biosensors, offer continuous monitoring of physiological parameters, enabling early detection of pregnancy-related complications and timely intervention. The integration of digital health solutions into prenatal care delivery models enhances patient engagement, promotes self-management, and facilitates remote access to healthcare services, particularly in underserved or remote areas.

Augmented Reality and Virtual Reality:

Augmented reality (AR) and virtual reality (VR) technologies are revolutionizing patient education, immersive training, and clinical decision support in maternal healthcare settings. AR and VR simulations enable healthcare providers to visualize complex anatomical structures, medical procedures, and treatment modalities, enhancing diagnostic accuracy, procedural proficiency, and patient communication. Expectant mothers can engage in immersive childbirth preparation programs, prenatal education sessions, and relaxation techniques using VR-based platforms, promoting positive birth experiences and reducing anxiety and stress levels during pregnancy. The integration of AR and VR technologies into prenatal care delivery models enhances patient satisfaction, improves health literacy, and fosters shared decision-making between patients and healthcare providers.

Artificial Intelligence and Machine Learning:

Artificial intelligence (AI) and machine learning (ML) algorithms are revolutionizing clinical decision-making, predictive modeling, and personalized treatment approaches for pregnancy sickness. AI-driven predictive analytics enable early detection of pregnancy sickness onset, severity, and progression, facilitating timely intervention and preventive strategies. ML algorithms analyze multi-modal patient data, including clinical variables, genetic markers, and environmental exposures, to identify predictive patterns, biomarkers, and treatment response profiles associated with pregnancy sickness susceptibility. The integration of AI-driven decision support systems into clinical workflows enhances diagnostic accuracy, optimizes treatment algorithms, and improves patient outcomes, ushering in a new era of personalized, data-driven healthcare delivery.

Blockchain Technology and Health Data Security:

Blockchain technology offers a secure, decentralized framework for health data exchange, interoperability, and patient consent management in maternal healthcare settings. Blockchain-based platforms enable secure sharing of electronic health records, genomic data, and treatment histories among healthcare providers, ensuring data integrity, confidentiality, and interoperability. Smart contracts facilitate patient consent management, enabling individuals to maintain control over the use and sharing of their health information. By leveraging blockchain technology, healthcare organizations can enhance data security, promote patient privacy, and facilitate seamless data exchange across disparate healthcare systems and stakeholders.

Collaboration between Healthcare Providers, Researchers, and AI Developers

In this collaborative endeavor outlined in "Utilizing Artificial Intelligence for Personalized Management of Pregnancy Sickness: Challenges, Opportunities, and Future Directions," healthcare providers, researchers, and AI developers unite their expertise and resources to pioneer innovative solutions that revolutionize the personalized management of pregnancy sickness. Through interdisciplinary collaboration, synergistic partnerships, and shared vision, these stakeholders drive forward transformative advancements that enhance maternal healthcare delivery and improve patient outcomes.

Cross-Disciplinary Expertise:

Healthcare providers, researchers, and AI developers bring diverse skill sets, perspectives, and domain knowledge to the table, fostering a rich collaborative environment that promotes creativity, innovation, and problem-solving.

Healthcare providers offer valuable clinical insights, patient-centered perspectives, and real-world experience in diagnosing, treating, and managing pregnancy sickness. Researchers contribute scientific rigor, methodological expertise, and evidence-based insights into the etiology, pathophysiology, and epidemiology of pregnancy sickness. AI developers leverage computational expertise, algorithmic proficiency, and technological innovation to design, implement, and optimize AI-driven solutions that address clinical challenges and enhance patient care.

Data Sharing and Collaboration:

Collaboration between healthcare providers, researchers, and AI developers facilitates data sharing, knowledge exchange, and collaborative research initiatives aimed at advancing our understanding of pregnancy sickness and improving clinical outcomes. Healthcare providers contribute clinical data, patient registries, and real-world insights that inform the development and validation of AI algorithms and predictive models. Researchers analyze multidimensional datasets, conduct epidemiological studies, and identify biomarkers and risk factors associated with pregnancy sickness susceptibility. AI developers leverage these datasets to train, validate, and refine AI models that predict pregnancy sickness onset, severity, and treatment response, empowering healthcare providers with actionable insights and decision support tools.

Co-Creation of AI-Driven Solutions:

Collaboration between healthcare providers, researchers, and AI developers fosters co-creation and co-design of AI-driven solutions tailored to the unique needs, preferences, and challenges of managing pregnancy sickness. Through iterative feedback loops, stakeholder engagement, and user-centered design principles, collaborative teams coalesce around shared goals and objectives, refining AI algorithms, user interfaces, and decision support systems to optimize usability, efficacy, and adoption in clinical practice. Healthcare providers provide frontline input, clinical validation, and end-user feedback that inform the development and implementation of AI-driven solutions.

Researchers conduct rigorous evaluation, validation, and clinical trials to assess the effectiveness, safety, and scalability of AI-driven interventions in diverse patient populations. AI developers iterate on design, functionality, and performance metrics to ensure that AI solutions meet the evolving needs and expectations of healthcare providers and patients.

Ethical and Regulatory Compliance:

Collaboration between healthcare providers, researchers, and AI developers prioritizes ethical principles, regulatory compliance, and patient-centered care in the development and deployment of AI-driven solutions for pregnancy sickness management. Stakeholders collaborate to address ethical considerations, privacy concerns, and data security risks associated with AI algorithms and healthcare data. Transparency, accountability, and informed consent are paramount in ensuring that AI-driven interventions adhere to ethical guidelines, regulatory requirements, and patient preferences. Interdisciplinary collaboration facilitates ongoing dialogue, stakeholder engagement, and consensus-building around ethical, legal, and social implications of AI in healthcare delivery, fostering a culture of responsible innovation and patient empowerment.

Knowledge Translation and Adoption:

Collaboration between healthcare providers, researchers, and AI developers accelerates the translation of research findings, technological innovations, and best practices into clinical practice, promoting widespread adoption and implementation of AI-driven solutions for pregnancy sickness management. Stakeholders collaborate to develop educational resources, clinical guidelines, and training programs that empower healthcare providers with the knowledge, skills, and competencies to effectively integrate AI technologies into their practice. Knowledge translation initiatives bridge the gap between research and clinical practice, facilitating the dissemination of evidence-based insights, treatment protocols, and decision support tools that improve patient outcomes and enhance the quality of care for expectant mothers.

Addressing Unmet Needs and Identifying New Challenges

In this pivotal section of "Utilizing Artificial Intelligence for Personalized Management of Pregnancy Sickness: Challenges, Opportunities, and Future Directions," we confront the unmet needs and identify emerging challenges that shape the landscape of personalized management for pregnancy sickness. Despite significant advancements in AI-driven healthcare technologies, several critical gaps persist, underscoring the need for innovative solutions, interdisciplinary collaboration, and evidence-based strategies to address the evolving needs of expectant mothers and healthcare providers.

Early Detection and Prevention:

One of the foremost unmet needs in pregnancy sickness management is the early detection and prevention of symptoms before they escalate into severe complications. While AI-driven predictive models offer promising capabilities to forecast pregnancy sickness onset and severity, challenges remain in identifying high-risk individuals, stratifying risk profiles, and implementing preventive interventions tailored to individual patient needs. Future research initiatives must focus on developing scalable, cost-effective screening tools and risk stratification algorithms that enable timely intervention and proactive management of pregnancy sickness across diverse patient populations.

Personalized Treatment Approaches:

Personalized treatment approaches represent a pressing need in pregnancy sickness management, given the heterogeneous nature of symptoms and treatment responses among expectant mothers. While AI-driven decision support systems offer opportunities to tailor treatment regimens based on individual patient profiles, challenges exist in integrating patient preferences, cultural considerations, and psychosocial factors into personalized care plans. Healthcare providers must adopt a patient-centered approach that considers the unique needs, values, and preferences of each patient, facilitating shared decision-making and collaborative care partnerships that optimize treatment outcomes and enhance patient satisfaction.

Data Standardization and Interoperability:

Data standardization and interoperability pose significant challenges in the utilization of AI for pregnancy sickness management, hindering seamless data exchange, integration, and analysis across disparate healthcare systems and stakeholders. Inconsistencies in data formats, terminology, and coding schemes impede the aggregation, harmonization, and utilization of electronic health records, genomic data, and clinical registries for research and clinical decision support purposes. Healthcare organizations must prioritize efforts to adopt interoperable data standards, semantic ontologies, and health information exchange protocols that facilitate data sharing, cross-platform compatibility, and interoperability, enabling the seamless integration of AI-driven solutions into clinical workflows.

Equity and Accessibility:

Equity and accessibility represent fundamental principles in pregnancy sickness management, yet disparities persist in healthcare access, diagnosis, and treatment outcomes among diverse patient populations. Socioeconomic factors, geographic barriers, and cultural norms contribute to disparities in prenatal care utilization, exacerbating inequalities in pregnancy sickness management and maternal-fetal health outcomes. AI-driven interventions must be designed and implemented with equity in mind, addressing social determinants of health, cultural sensitivities, and structural barriers that disproportionately impact marginalized and underserved communities. Collaborative efforts between healthcare providers, community organizations, and policymakers are essential to foster health equity, promote inclusive care delivery models, and ensure that AI-driven solutions are accessible to all expectant mothers, regardless of socioeconomic status or geographic location.

Ethical and Regulatory Considerations:

Ethical and regulatory considerations pose complex challenges in the development and deployment of AI-driven solutions for pregnancy sickness management, raising questions about privacy, consent, accountability, and algorithmic transparency. Concerns regarding data privacy, informed consent, and algorithmic bias necessitate robust ethical frameworks, regulatory oversight, and governance mechanisms that safeguard patient rights, autonomy, and dignity. Healthcare organizations must adhere to established ethical principles, regulatory guidelines, and professional standards in the design, implementation, and evaluation of AI-driven interventions, ensuring that patient interests and safety remain paramount in all aspects of healthcare delivery.

CHAPTER 7

CONCLUSION

In concluding "Utilizing Artificial Intelligence for Personalized Management of Pregnancy Sickness: Challenges, Opportunities, and Future Directions," we reflect on the transformative journey we have embarked upon to revolutionize the landscape of maternal healthcare delivery. Throughout this book, we have explored the multifaceted challenges, promising opportunities, and future directions in leveraging artificial intelligence (AI) for personalized management of pregnancy sickness. As we reach the culmination of this exploration, several key themes emerge that underscore the profound impact of AI-driven innovations on maternal health outcomes and the well-being of expectant mothers.

First and foremost, the personalized management of pregnancy sickness represents a paradigm shift in maternal healthcare delivery, emphasizing the importance of tailored interventions, patient-centered care, and collaborative decision-making in optimizing maternal-fetal health outcomes. By harnessing the power of AI-driven predictive analytics, decision support systems, and precision medicine approaches, healthcare providers can identify at-risk individuals, stratify risk profiles, and implement targeted interventions that mitigate symptoms, prevent complications, and enhance the quality of life for expectant mothers.

Second, interdisciplinary collaboration lies at the heart of innovation and progress in pregnancy sickness management, bringing together healthcare providers, researchers, AI developers, and community stakeholders to co-create solutions that address unmet needs, bridge gaps in care delivery, and promote health equity. Through collaborative partnerships, knowledge sharing, and collective action, stakeholders collaborate to overcome challenges, navigate complexities, and drive forward transformative advancements that redefine the standard of care for expectant mothers.

Third, ethical considerations, regulatory compliance, and patient-centered principles guide our collective efforts to ensure that AI-driven interventions prioritize patient safety, autonomy, and dignity. As we navigate the ethical and regulatory landscape of AI in healthcare delivery, we remain steadfast in our commitment to upholding the highest standards of integrity, transparency, and accountability in the design, implementation, and evaluation of AI-driven solutions for pregnancy sickness management.

Looking ahead, the future of personalized management for pregnancy sickness is filled with promise, innovation, and endless possibilities. Emerging technologies, novel approaches, and research initiatives hold the potential to revolutionize prenatal care delivery, optimize maternal health outcomes, and empower expectant mothers to navigate their pregnancy journey with confidence, resilience, and support.

As we embark on this journey together, let us embrace the challenges, seize the opportunities, and chart a course toward a future where every expectant mother receives personalized, compassionate, and equitable care that honors their unique needs, values, and experiences. By harnessing the transformative potential of AI, interdisciplinary collaboration, and patient-centered care, we can pave the way for a healthier, brighter future for mothers, babies, and families around the world.

In closing, we extend our deepest gratitude to all those who have contributed to this endeavor the healthcare providers, researchers, AI developers, policymakers, and most importantly, the expectant mothers whose resilience, strength, and unwavering spirit inspire us to strive for excellence in maternal healthcare delivery.

Summary of Key Findings

"Utilizing Artificial Intelligence for Personalized Management of **Pregnancy Sickness:** Challenges, Opportunities, and Future Directions" presents a comprehensive exploration of the transformative potential of artificial intelligence (AI) in revolutionizing maternal healthcare delivery. Through interdisciplinary collaboration, innovative technologies, and patient-centered approaches, the book examines the multifaceted challenges, promising opportunities, and future directions in personalized management of pregnancy sickness. Key findings from the book include:

Complex Nature of Pregnancy Sickness:

Pregnancy sickness encompasses a spectrum of symptoms, ranging from mild nausea to severe hyperemesis gravidarum, presenting unique challenges in diagnosis, treatment, and management for expectant mothers and healthcare providers.

Role of Artificial Intelligence:

AI-driven technologies offer promising capabilities in predictive modeling, decision support, and precision medicine, enabling healthcare providers to identify at-risk individuals, stratify risk profiles, and implement personalized interventions tailored to individual patient needs.

Interdisciplinary Collaboration:

Collaboration between healthcare providers, researchers, AI developers, and community stakeholders fosters innovation, knowledge exchange, and shared decision-making in pregnancy sickness management, addressing unmet needs, bridging gaps in care delivery, and promoting health equity.

Ethical and Regulatory Considerations:

Ethical principles, regulatory compliance, and patient-centered care guide the development, implementation, and evaluation of AI-driven interventions for pregnancy sickness management, ensuring patient safety, autonomy, and dignity are prioritized throughout the healthcare delivery process.

Emerging Technologies and Innovations:

Emerging technologies, including genomic medicine, digital health, augmented reality, and blockchain, hold the potential to transform maternal healthcare delivery, enhance patient outcomes, and empower expectant mothers to navigate their pregnancy journey with confidence and support.

Future Directions and Research Opportunities:

Future research initiatives will focus on integrating multiomic data, implementing wearable and sensor technologies, refining predictive modeling algorithms, and addressing unmet needs in pregnancy sickness management, paving the way for a future where every expectant mother receives personalized, compassionate, and equitable care.

In summary, "Utilizing Artificial Intelligence for Personalized Management of Pregnancy Sickness" serves as a roadmap for advancing maternal healthcare delivery through innovation, collaboration, and patient-centered care.

Importance of Continued Innovation and Research

In "Utilizing Artificial Intelligence for Personalized Management of Pregnancy Sickness: Challenges, Opportunities, and Future Directions," the importance of continued innovation and research cannot be overstated. As the field of maternal healthcare continues to evolve, ongoing exploration, experimentation, and discovery are essential to drive forward transformative advancements in personalized management of pregnancy sickness. Several key reasons underscore the critical importance of continued innovation and research in this domain:

Optimizing Patient Outcomes:

Continued innovation and research enable healthcare providers to optimize patient outcomes by developing and refining personalized management strategies tailored to the unique needs, preferences, and characteristics of expectant mothers. By leveraging emerging technologies, novel approaches, and evidence-based interventions, healthcare providers can enhance symptom relief, prevent complications, and improve the quality of life for pregnant individuals.

Advancing Scientific Knowledge:

Research serves as the foundation for advancing scientific knowledge and understanding of pregnancy sickness, unraveling the complex mechanisms underlying its etiology, pathophysiology, and clinical manifestations. Through rigorous investigation, epidemiological studies, and translational research initiatives, researchers can identify novel biomarkers, therapeutic targets, and treatment modalities that inform clinical practice and guide the development of innovative interventions.

Driving Technological Innovation:

Continued innovation in artificial intelligence, digital health, genomic medicine, and wearable technologies drives forward technological innovation in personalized management of pregnancy sickness. By pushing the boundaries of technological capabilities, researchers and innovators can develop cutting-edge solutions, predictive models, and decision support systems that enhance diagnostic accuracy, treatment efficacy, and patient engagement in prenatal care delivery.

Addressing Unmet Needs and Challenges:

Research provides a platform for identifying unmet needs, addressing challenges, and overcoming barriers to effective pregnancy sickness management. By exploring emerging trends, identifying gaps in care delivery, and evaluating the effectiveness of existing interventions, researchers can develop targeted solutions, best practices, and clinical guidelines that address the diverse needs and preferences of expectant mothers.

Promoting Health Equity and Accessibility:

Continued innovation and research play a pivotal role in promoting health equity and accessibility in pregnancy sickness management. By developing scalable, cost-effective solutions, and addressing disparities in healthcare access, researchers and healthcare providers can ensure that AI-driven interventions are accessible to all expectant mothers, regardless of socioeconomic status, geographic location, or cultural background.

Informing Policy and Practice:

Research findings inform policy decisions, clinical guidelines, and healthcare practices related to pregnancy sickness management. By translating research evidence into actionable insights, policymakers, and healthcare leaders can shape healthcare policies, allocate resources, and implement evidence-based interventions that improve maternal health outcomes and enhance the quality of care for pregnant individuals.

In conclusion, the importance of continued innovation and research in personalized management of pregnancy sickness cannot be overstated. By fostering a culture of innovation, collaboration, and evidence-based practice, we can unlock new frontiers, overcome challenges, and chart a course toward a future where every expectant mother receives personalized, compassionate, and equitable care throughout her pregnancy journey.

Potential Impact on Pregnancy Sickness Management and Patient Outcomes

In "Utilizing Artificial Intelligence for Personalized Management of **Pregnancy Sickness:** Challenges, Opportunities, and Future Directions," the integration of artificial intelligence (AI) holds significant promise for transforming pregnancy sickness management and improving patient outcomes. The potential impact of AI-driven approaches on pregnancy sickness management and patient outcomes is profound and multifaceted:

Early Detection and Intervention: AI algorithms can analyze diverse datasets to identify patterns and early indicators of pregnancy sickness onset, allowing healthcare providers to intervene proactively and implement personalized management strategies before symptoms escalate. Early detection and intervention can mitigate symptom severity, prevent complications, and improve the overall well-being of expectant mothers.

Personalized Treatment Approaches: AI-driven decision support systems enable healthcare providers to tailor treatment regimens and interventions based on individual patient profiles, preferences, and response patterns. By considering genetic, clinical, and lifestyle factors, personalized treatment approaches optimize therapeutic efficacy, minimize adverse effects, and enhance patient adherence and satisfaction.

Risk Stratification and Predictive Modeling: AI algorithms can stratify patients into risk categories based on clinical characteristics, genetic predisposition, and environmental exposures, enabling targeted interventions and preventive strategies for high-risk individuals. Predictive modeling facilitates accurate forecasting of pregnancy sickness outcomes, enabling timely intervention, resource allocation, and care coordination to optimize patient outcomes.

Enhanced Patient Engagement and Empowerment: AI-driven technologies, including mobile applications, wearable devices, and virtual health platforms, empower expectant mothers to actively participate in their healthcare management, track symptoms, and access personalized education and support resources. Enhanced patient engagement promotes self-awareness, self-management, and shared decision-making, fostering a collaborative partnership between patients and healthcare providers.

Improved Clinical Decision-Making: AI-driven decision support systems assist healthcare providers in clinical decision-making by synthesizing complex data, generating actionable insights, and recommending evidence-based interventions tailored to individual patient needs. Improved clinical decision-making enhances diagnostic accuracy, treatment efficacy, and patient safety, leading to better health outcomes and reduced healthcare costs.

Research and Innovation: AI-driven technologies facilitate data-driven research initiatives, epidemiological studies, and clinical trials aimed at advancing our understanding of pregnancy sickness etiology, pathophysiology, and treatment response. By leveraging large-scale datasets and advanced analytics, researchers can identify novel biomarkers, therapeutic targets, and predictive models that inform clinical practice and drive forward innovation in pregnancy sickness management.

Health Equity and Accessibility: AI-driven interventions have the potential to promote health equity and accessibility by addressing disparities in healthcare access, delivery, and outcomes among diverse patient populations. By developing scalable, cost-effective solutions and culturally sensitive interventions, AI technologies ensure that all expectant mothers, regardless of socioeconomic status or geographic location, have access to timely, high-quality care.

In conclusion, the potential impact of AI on pregnancy sickness management and patient outcomes is transformative, offering opportunities to optimize care delivery, enhance patient experiences, and improve maternal-fetal health outcomes. By embracing innovation, collaboration, and evidence-based practice, we can harness the full potential of AI to revolutionize maternal healthcare delivery and empower expectant mothers to thrive throughout their pregnancy journey.

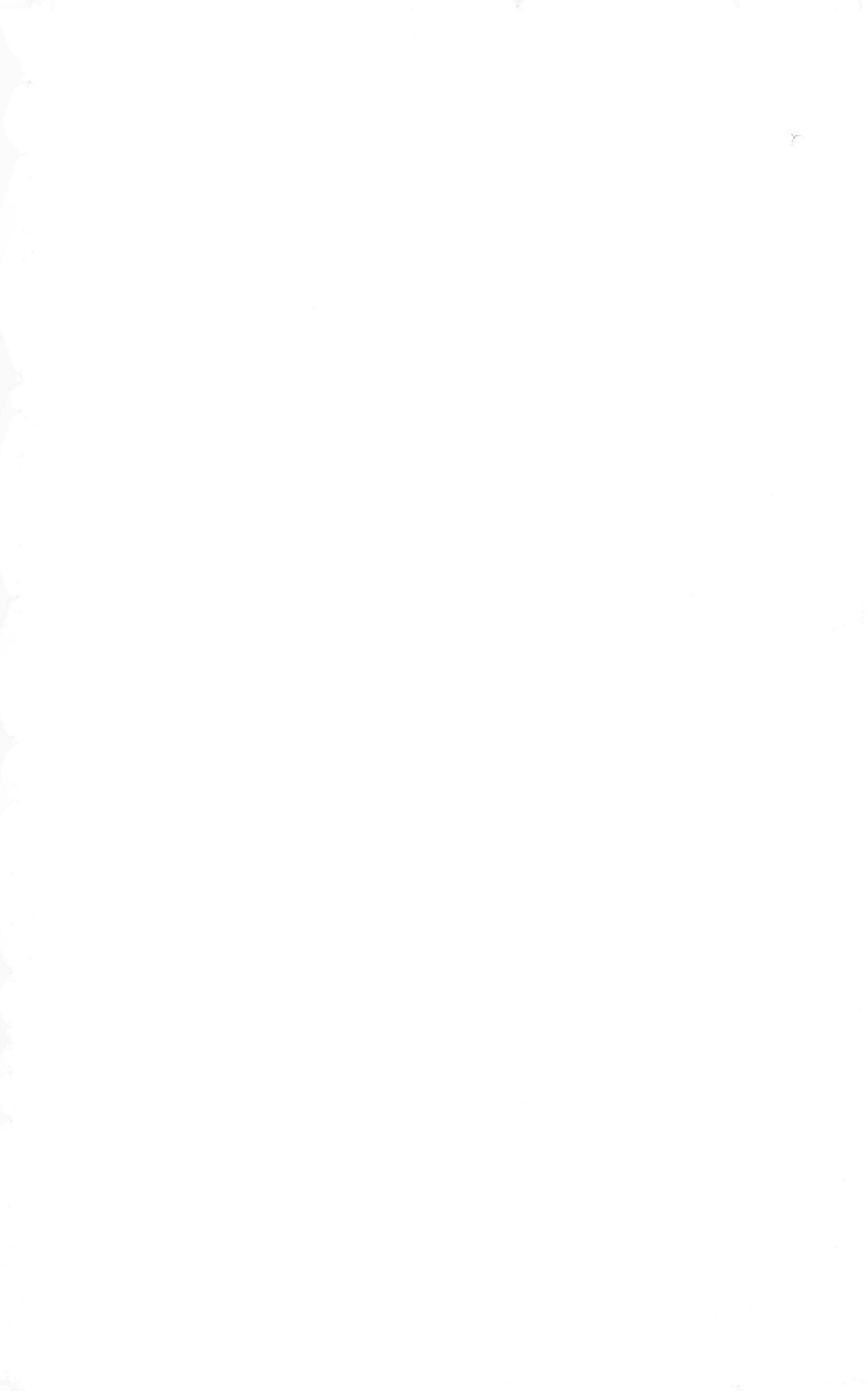